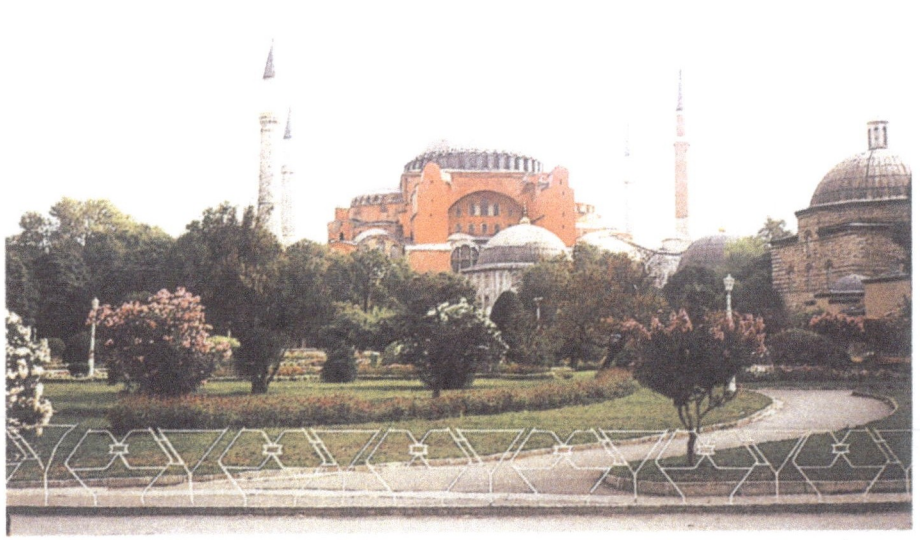

Are the medical needs for the treatment of acute pain fulfilled?

Istanbul, Turkey, October 5, 1996

Springer Basel AG

A CIP catalogue record for this book is available from the Library of Congress, Washington, D.C., USA

Deutsche Bibliothek – Cataloging-in-Publication Data

Are the medical needs for the treatment of acute pain fulfilled? : Istanbul, Turkey, October 5th, 1996 – Springer Basel AG
ISBN 978-3-7643-5679-8   ISBN 978-3-0348-8867-7 (eBook)
DOI 10.1007/978-3-0348-8867-7

1997 Springer Basel AG
Originally published by Birkhäuser Verlag in 1997
Printed on acid-free paper produced from chlorine-free pulp. TCF ∞

ISBN 978-3-7643-5679-8

9 8 7 6 5 4 3 2 1

Contents

Introduction

Many effective analgesic drugs are available for the relief of acute pain, but their clinical use is widely regarded as being inadequate. The reasons cited for this include concern about the adverse effects of opioids and also insufficient adjustment of therapy to the patient´s needs. Non-opioid analgesics are the staple drugs for mild to moderate pain and are generally better tolerated than opioid drugs. Differences exist, however, among the non-opioid analgesics which affect the choice of drug for individual patients and specific acutely painful conditions.

In an associated symposium of the 7th International Symposium: The Pain Clinic, held in Istanbul, Turkey, the ways were discussed in which treatment with non-opioid analgesics can be tailored to meet the needs of individual patients with acute pain. The highlights of this Hoechst symposium, emphasize the distinctions between the non-steroidal anti-inflammatory drugs, and the non-acidic antipyretic analgesics, particularly dipyrone.

Mechanisms of action of non-opioid analgesics

Professor F.C. Tulunay, M.D.
Ankara, Turkey

The non-opioid analgesics are among the oldest class of synthetic drugs still in widespread clinical use. They can be divided into the non-steroidal anti-inflammatory drugs (NSAIDs), such as acetylsalicylic acid, and the non-acidic, antipyretic analgesics, paracetamol and dipyrone. The pharmacology of these various agents will be reviewed briefly.

The major mechanism of action of NSAIDs, proposed by Vane in 1971, is the inhibition of cycloxygenase (COX), the enzyme catalysing the synthesis of prostaglandins (PGs). Since PGE_2 has inflammatory, hyperalgesic and fever-inducing actions, inhibition of its synthesis explains the anti-inflammatory, analgesic and antipyretic properties of NSAIDs. Inhibition of the protective effects of PGE_2 on the gastric mucosa also helps explain the gastrointestinal (GI) side-effects of NSAIDs. It is now known that there is a constitutive enzyme (COX-1) producing PGs with a physiological role and another enzyme, COX-2, which is induced at inflamed sites. Most NSAIDs inhibit both enzymes.

Paracetamol and dipyrone, however, are very weak inhibitors of COX-1/COX-2 and are therefore devoid of anti-inflammatory activity, but have less GI side-effects than the NSAIDs. The anti-pyretic actions of both groups of drugs appear to be related to inhibition of PG synthesis in the brain, possibly through an action on a third COX isoenzyme. The analgesic effects of dipyrone and paracetamol are also mediated by central nervous system actions, which are as yet undefined.

"Dipyrone (though) a weak prostaglandin synthesis inhibitor, prevents hyperalgesia and down-regulates pain receptors."

Most NSAIDs are acidic, a property which contributes to their accumulation at inflamed sites and also within the gastric mucosa. NSAIDs with longer plasma half-lives show improved clinical compliance, but are also associated with a higher incidence of GI side-effects. Adverse hepatic, renal and allergic events also occur in response to NSAIDs. The incidence of adverse events to the non-acidic analgesics, on the other hand, is much lower, because of their different pattern of accumulation which includes access to the central nervous system.

Dipyrone is a pro-drug, being metabolized to the active metabolites, 4-methylaminoantipyrine and 4-aminoantipyrine. It is at least comparable to NSAIDs in its relief of acute pain and has the added advantage of an intrinsic spasmolytic action, making dipyrone particularly effective in renal and biliary colic pain (Fig. 1). In these indications, dipyrone has a rapid onset of action.

In conclusion, the efficacy of the versatile analgesic dipyrone has been demonstrated in a variety of acutely painful conditions, including pain following dental, abdominal and orthopedic surgery.

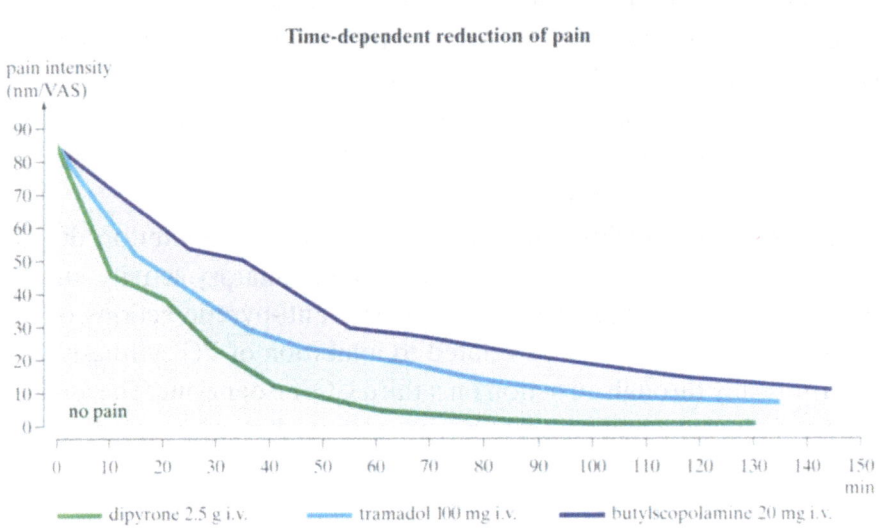

Fig. 1:
Comparative efficacy of parenteral dipyrone and other treatments in biliary colic patients.
VAS = visual analogue scale.
(Schmieder, G. et al., Arzneim. Forsch./Drug Res. 43 (II), No. 11, 1216–1221, 1993)

Fulfilling patients' needs for appropriate prescriptions: The acute pain service approach

P.F. Bejarano, M.D.
Bogota, Columbia

Even though the most widely prescribed drugs for the relief of acute pain have been in use for many years, their efficacy can still be enhanced by more precise assessment of pain and the judicial titration of doses. Some of the procedures applied within the Acute Pain Service of the Fundation Santa Fe de Bogota, as an example of the way in which an integrated approach can improve analgesic drug efficacy, will be discussed here.

> "The issue of pain management is not just (a matter of) prescription (but also involves) the needs of the patient."

Following surgery, patient needs include immediate analgesia, minimal disability, no drug side-effects, the possibility of early oral food and drug intake, good sleep and a rapid return to normal mobility. In seeking to meet these needs, it must also be taken into account that pain and surgical stress increase metabolic rate and autonomic responses and decrease immunological surveillance. These changes demand the application of a complete peri-operative analgesia concept (Fig. 1) which adjusts pain management to different phases of hospitalization.

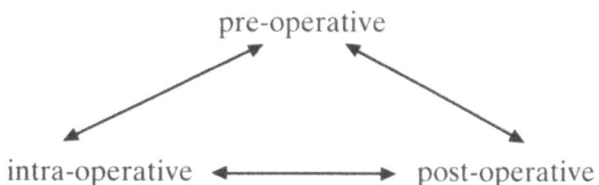

Fig. 1:
The peri-operative analgesia concept.

Pre-operatively, it is important to explain to the patient, using booklets and discussion, the sort of pain which might be expected and how it can be counteracted. In some cases, pre-emptive analgesia can be applied. Long-acting analgesics should be given before surgery, so that their optimal effects are achieved post-operatively.

In a 1988 survey of post-operative pain control in a clinical hospital setting, it was found that only 42.5% of patients had adequate pain control, even though 55% of them were receiving opioids. In as many as 73% of cases, analgesics were not prescribed according to recommendations. Because of a lack of understanding of physiology among physicians pain is often considered to be harmless and analgesia is given low priority; lack of understanding of pharmacology raises a fear of adverse effects leading to administration of inadequate analgesic doses; poor pain evaluation distracts attention from the patient's complaints and results in disregard of the patient's needs.

Not only is sufficient understanding of treatment measures and pain assessment required of the physician, there must also be an appreciation of the fact that various types of pain must be approached differently. Visceral pain can best be treated by reducing distension, while musculoskeletal pain usually requires anti-inflammatory analgesia. Non-steroidal anti-inflammatory drugs (NSAIDs), though, vary to some extent particularly in their pharmacokinetics; they act mainly to inhibit peripheral nociceptor sensitization and to prevent hyperalgesia. Dipyrone alone among non-opioid analgesics is able to inhibit ongoing hyperalgesia, probably by affecting synthesis of nitric oxide. In Bogota, intramuscular injection of dipyrone is avoided and the drug is given at a dose of 50 mg/kg i.v. to reduce potential side-effects.

A careful assessment of the risk of adverse events also contributes to the selection of the optimal analgesic, a decision which requires predetermination of post-operative analgesic goals. Therefore, better analgesics may not be required for treatment of acute pain, but rather improved integration of the measures which are currently available.

Non-opioids in the treatment of post-operative pain

Professor N. Rawal, M.D., Ph.D.
Örebro, Sweden

Routine post-operative pain relief is still considered to be inadequate. In a European survey of 17 countries, 55% of anesthesiologists in 105 hospitals were dissatisfied with pain treatment on surgical wards and a survey of 300 hospitals in the United States provided similar figures. The common technique of providing intramuscular opioids on a post-operative, "as-needed" basis is often insufficient and is also unrealistic in the face of the problem of pain at home after leaving the hospital. Non-opioid analgesics can play a major role in this situation.

Within the hospital setting, non-opioid analgesics are playing an increasingly important role in the multi-modal approach to post-operative pain management, which incorporates various drugs, routes of administration and organisation of pain services into the management plan.

Regional techniques avoid the hazards of sedation and in Örebro surgical wounds are routinely infiltrated with local anesthetic before suturing. This is simple, cheap and effective.

The usefulness of non-opioid analgesics in opioid-sparing therapy is questionable, because even with a reduction of the dose, adverse effects of opioids such as nausea, vomiting and sleep disturbances still occur. A better approach, where feasible, is to administer a non-opioid analgesic alone. In Örebro, 1g paracetamol, four times daily, is given as a basal medication. With the recent re-introduction to Sweden of the more potent dipyrone, it will be interesting to investigate the potential of this drug as a basal analgesic. A further advantage of using a non-opioid rather than an opioid for post-operative analgesia is that patients are able to eat and drink earlier, leading to a more rapid return to normal mobility.

"all non-opioids are not created equal."

As pointed out by other speakers, the differences among non-opioid analgesics should be emphasized. NSAIDs cause gastrointestinal disturbances and bleeding and may result in renal impairment. Ibuprofen use, however, is associated with a lower risk of bleeding than that of some other NSAIDs. Dipyrone use, on the other hand, is not associated with any risk of bleeding (Table 1).

Table 1:
Platelet function (mean values) after 3g dipyrone daily or placebo in male volunteers

| | Platelet count (x 10^9/l) | | Bleeding time (min) | |
	Placebo	Drug	Placebo	Drug
Day 1	221	212	6.07	6.38
Day 2	226	205	6.63	7.69

S.J. Machin & I.E. Mackie (1993) In: *Modern Principles in the Management of Pain.* Ed. L.J. de Souza et al, Hoechst India, Bombay, 1994.

In Örebro, great importance is placed on informing the patient pre-operatively about the pain management modalities which will be used. The patient is told that the visual analogue score for pain, taken every 3 h, will be kept below a score of three post-operatively. Intravenous opioids are administered when basal paracetamol medication and local anesthetic wound infiltration is insufficient.

In conclusion, non-opioids have a major role to play in post-operative pain management, both given systemically and by regional techniques. The fact that NSAIDs differ among themselves and from paracetamol and dipyrone in their properties highlights the importance of balancing the risks and benefits of individual drugs before selection for pain relief. There are no absolutely safe drugs, therefore, the emphasis should be placed on the best way to treat the pain.

Comparative safety of non-opioid analgesics

C. Martinez, M.D.
Frankfurt/Main, Germany

When considering the safety of non-opioid analgesics, particularly that of the non-steroidal anti-inflammatory drugs (NSAIDs), gastrointestinal side-effects spring most readily to mind. Actually, non-opioid analgesic use is associated with a variety of other adverse events, including renal, hepatic and blood cell effects. Because of the different nature of these adverse events they cannot normally be combined for an overall comparison of drug safety. Using death due to any serious adverse event as a common health outcome in a three-dimensional approach which includes the profile and frequency of adverse events, the overall safety of non-opioid analgesics can be compared.

A search of the literature from 1970 to 1995 revealed eleven cohort or case control studies in which the comparative risks among non-opioid analgesics of the occurrence of *potentially fatal* adverse events were assessed. These included seven studies on gastrointestinal complications and one each on agranulocytosis, aplastic anemia, anaphylaxis and Stevens-Johnson syndrome/toxic epidermal necrolysis (SJS/TEN), a response which leads to skin detachment. Four drugs (dipyrone, paracetamol, aspirin and diclofenac) were included in all these studies. The estimated frequency of death due to the five different adverse events was calculated.

In the total community the incidence of gastrointestinal bleeding disorders for all causes (310-1000 cases/10^6 per year) is much greater than that of the other disorders (e.g. agranulocytosis, 3.4 cases/10^6 per year). The likelihood of death from gastrointestinal bleeding resulting in hospitalization is 23–33% and 10% for agranulocytosis.

"Taking overall mortality due to different causes, (expected) mortality from dipyrone use is much lower than that from aspirin or diclofenac."

This incidence profile is also reflected in the overall expected mortality which was attributed to the various non-opioid analgesics (Fig. 1). It is immediately apparent that gastrointestinal complications are responsible for the overwhelming majority of overall expected deaths due to use of any analgesic. Moreover, use of NSAIDs is associated with a much higher risk of death due to gastrointestinal complications and to adverse events overall than is the use of a non-acidic analgesic such as dipyrone. While 57.5 deaths/million users due to adverse events can be expected on azapropazone treatment, the figure is 1.9 for aspirin use and only 0.2 for dipyrone. It is worth noting that with 0.039 expected deaths due to agranulocytosis per million users of dipyrone (18% of all expected deaths on dipyrone) the risk of death by this cause would have to be several orders of magnitude greater before being comparable with the risk of death due to aspirin use. Furthermore, idiosyncratic reactions such as agranulocytosis and anaphylaxis are less likely on oral than on parenteral administration.

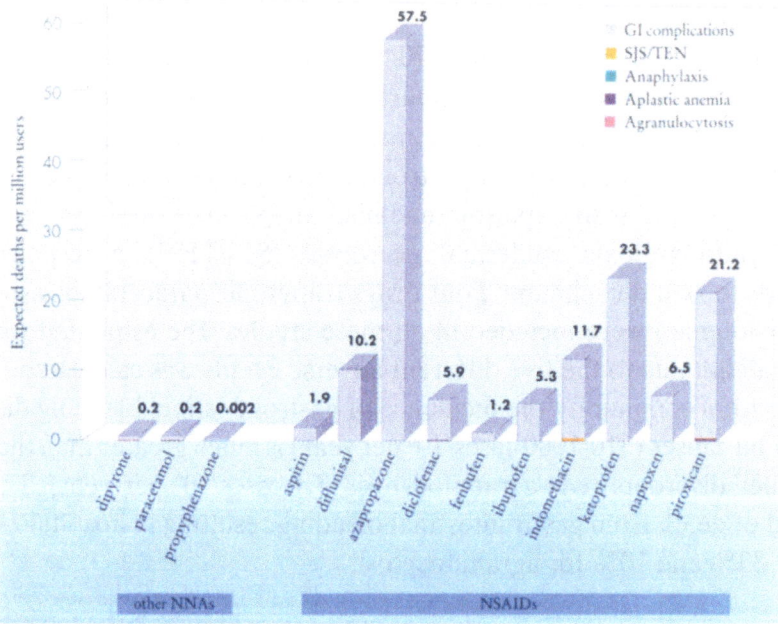

Fig. 1:
Overall mortality per million users expected on administration of various non-opioid analgesics for one week (NNAs = non-narcotic analgesics, NSAIDs = non-steroidal anti-inflammatory drugs).

These data clearly show that because of the greater risk of gastrointestinal complications with short-term NSAID administration, the non-acidic analgesics, dipyrone and paracetamol, can be considered to be much safer. In comparison to gastrointestinal disorders, the risk of death due to other adverse events of non-opioid analgesics is very low.

Concluding remarks

A variety of analgesic drugs are available for the treatment of acute pain, but some are still inappropriately employed. The introduction of acute pain services considerably enhances the usefulness of the available analgesics. An important factor in the choice of analgesic is to ensure acceptable tolerability by the patient. In this respect, administration of dipyrone has the advantage of not being associated with the bleeding and gastrointestinal side-effects seen with NSAIDs. In addition, it lacks the typical adverse opioid effects, such as nausea, constipation and respiratory depression. Epidemiological studies show that dipyrone use carries a very low risk of serious side-effects. With its additional intrinsic spasmolytic properties, dipyrone helps to meet the medical need in the treatment of acute pain as a well-tolerated, potent, non-opioid analgesic.

GPSR Compliance

The European Union's (EU) General Product Safety Regulation (GPSR) is a set of rules that requires consumer products to be safe and our obligations to ensure this.

If you have any concerns about our products, you can contact us on ProductSafety@springernature.com

In case Publisher is established outside the EU, the EU authorized representative is:

Springer Nature Customer Service Center GmbH
Europaplatz 3
69115 Heidelberg, Germany

Batch number: 09636724

Printed by Printforce, the Netherlands